MW01125487

Everything you want to know about Japanese bondage. Guide in pictures.

Seito Saiki

Table of Contents

Disclaimer

While all attempts have been made to verify the information provided in this book, the author does assume any responsibility for errors, omissions, or contrary interpretations of the subject matter contained within. The information provided in this book is for educational and entertainment purposes only. The reader is responsible for his or her own actions and the author does not accept any responsibilities for any liabilities or damages, real or perceived, resulting from the use of this information.

The trademarks that are used are without any consent, and the publication of the trademark is without permission or backing by the trademark owner. All trademarks and brands within this book are for clarifying purposes only and are the owned by the owners themselves, not affiliated with this document.

Introduction

Welcome to the beginners guide to Shibari. In this book you will learn about what it takes to safely and confidently perform the Japanese art of Shibari otherwise known as bondage. The secret here is that not all bondage is sexual in nature. While it is obviously associated with that as well, it is also independently considered an art form and is practiced by very serious artists. The main difference is being in the word chosen to describe it. The word Shibari in Japanese is specific to the act of tying, or binding. Whereas Kinbaku is the more sexual side of it, the word associated the BDSM and sex games side of things. If you are referring to a beautiful artistic display that, while erotic, is limited to an artist's interpretation and not a sex act then you would be speaking of Shibari.

It is important to create that distinction in your mind early on to avoid any misconstruing of information or misleading of thoughts. While they are similar in a vast amount of ways, they are also incredibly different and specific to the art form that either one represents. It is not something to be taken lightly in sense of activity. It is altogether physically as well as emotionally involved. In this book specifically, we will go over some of the history of the art form and then delve into the actual practice of it. For instance, we will outline the materials you will need in order to actually perform it. Then we will actually break it down step by step with some basic introductory elements. From there, you will effectively learn how to take your first steps down the artistic road of Shibari bondage. You will in no way become an expert from reading this book as the art form takes much practice and concentration, but if you're just starting out and wondering how you could ever possibly start out and enjoy it, then this book is perfect for you. The fundamentals, basics and history, are all within these pages.

Not to mention that this is the perfect foundation to lay down for yourself when getting into something as complex and rewarding as this specific art form. Without taking up to much more of your time, knowing that you're looking to get started, lets end this introduction and move on into the history of Shibari itself so you can learn and expand the horizons with which you gaze upon it.

What is Shibari?

Perhaps you got this book as a gift from someone who thought you might be interested, or perhaps you read about it somewhere and decided that this was the book you needed. Either way, you're reading this because you're intrigued. One of the best ways to get invested in something that intrigues you is to learn a bit about it. For instance, Shibari originates from as early as the 1400's in Japan. It was utilized by the highly renowned and revered Samurai. The art form started out as a form of restraining and restricting the prisoners of the Samurai originally known as Hojo-jutsu. For if you were a captive of Samurai it was considered to be an honorable thing, and they showed that even through the way you were restrained. From there it evolved and changed into the more expressive style of Shibari which is considered a vastly acceptable art form used by a wide variety of artists. This change was much more deeply noticeable in the early 1900's, when the art form took a decidedly more erotic turn in the way of a sensual and artistic representation and exposure. From there it has been taken even further into the regions of the aforementioned Kinbaku and from there on you could fall deep into the rabbit hole of the specifics.

Shibari is something that should be viewed as a multi-layered performance piece. For instance, it isn't just all about the rope. A huge part of it is the model herself/himself, and the way they are positioned. With there being realistically millions of different ways to achieve this, it becomes an infinitely expressive and interpretive art form that can be used to represent anything your brain can conceive. This practice is also something used with willing participants and is not considered to be synonymous with any form of deprivation or degradation; in fact it is quite the opposite. It is incredibly common for the models to experience a sort of high, or even a trance like state for the one who is tied up. While the person is handling them, also known as a rigger, can experience adrenaline highs from being in control. All this is from tying knots? Yes, but it also so much more than that.

The ability to tell a story and construct an artistic representation is represented by Shibari for ages now and it is becoming more and more popular in today's day in age as people look for different forms of expression. Ways to capture who they really are. It comes down to the body of the model and the way the ropes are arranged and the places the knots are tied. How the ropes compliment the curves of the body or how the knots accentuate the complexities of the body. There are so many individual elements that working together to create a beautiful display that captures your eyes and gives you something to think about.

In terms of back stories this art form has a rich one, rooted in a history of a culture so full of artistic revery and beauty. Without appreciating that you would be unable to proceed into crafting your own works of art confidently and with the respect required. Now that you have a basic understanding of its history, it's time to start taking a look at what we need in order to take our first steps in performing this art!

Materials for the Japanese art of Shibari

With as much as you know about the art form already, it is most likely safe to assume that you understand the main ingredient in the practicing of this ancient trade. If it hasn't made itself more apparent to you then allow me to shed light. You'll need rope.

This however is much easier to say than it is to do, only in the sense of specificity. Not just any rope will do. What you need is a rope that is specifically designed to be comfortable and to not cause pain or harm to your model. For instance, a cotton rope is one that is commonly used. However the most common and widely regarded are as best possible choice for this activity, it's something known as Jute rope. What that is, simply put, is a type of hemp rope made of natural materials. This is also another stipulation of respecting the trade. A demand made of most people to foray into the art form is that an all natural ingredient based rope is the greatest desired due to the traditional nature of the culture.

You can however utilize ropes that are made of more synthetic material as well if you would like. That is entirely up to your choice at the end of the day. What is important however you use ropes that are softer and pliable to your needs? In regards to the natural Jute rope, the fibers themselves make an excellent choice because the rope tends to cling to itself much nicer and stick together through the friction in twisting and turning or the knotting which makes for a much sturdier production. Another aspect to consider is length. In Japan the traditional length rounds out to around 24 feet. However in the western-most countries you would consider something closer to 28 feet based on the height difference. A small factor is to take into consideration when moving forward in this act.

As well, another thing to take in to consideration is the style of tying and binding that you intend to do. Including but not limited to whether or not you plan to suspend your model in the air, or keep them static on the ground. Certain cotton-like ropes are more delicate and wouldn't prove to be helpful in suspension, however synthetic is stronger. Although in terms of static scenarios cotton could be considered to be more comfortable than synthetic. A lot of your rope needs are to be laid out in the plan for the actual desired full effect early on in the production.

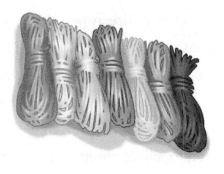

Knotting and Tying

Now we start to get into the actual fun part of the book. This is when we start to actually take a look at the different styles of knotting and tying that you will encounter as well as some of the techniques you can utilize in both of those tasks. The idea is to make it easy for you to understand and be able to follow along, so there will be pictures to assist in the creation of your own knots and ties. The goal with this main section of the book is to demonstrate a few lessons in which you can take away skills to eventually start practicing your own ties and knots. This tying and knotting is the core and central theme of Shibari. The display and how you present the art that you create is up to you, though we will touch on that a little bit at the end of this section here. Without further ado let's start getting into the different ways to tie up your model!

Below are a few examples of different basic knot techniques that you may encounter throughout the main section of the book.

BUTTERFLY KNOT

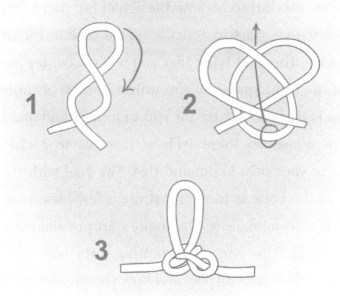

CONSTRICTOR CNOT

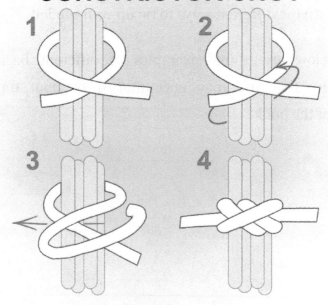

DOUBLE FISHERMANS

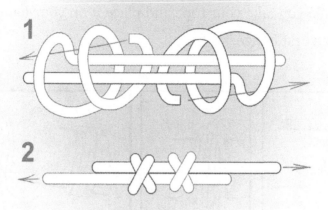

1

2

SLIP KNOT

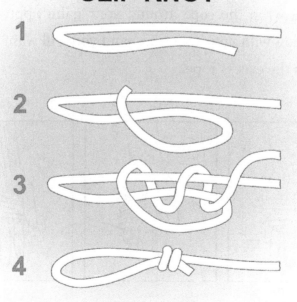

1

2

3

4

Hand tying "stirrup"

For this first one that we're going to do we are going to start simple. So you take your rope and place it on your hand as you see in the first image.

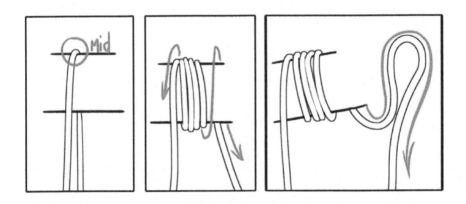

Then you wrap the rope around your palm approximately 5 times. Then with your opposite hand you will want to create a loop with the excess rope.

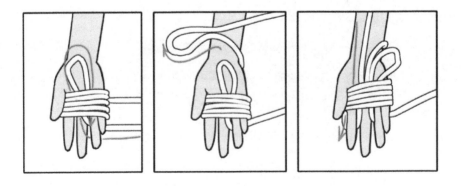

Then you will want to feed that extra loop under the coil you've created around your palm. Then you will take another loop and have it Bough up under your palm across from the other loop in your palm. Put that loop through the coil next to your other loop and between your two fingers.

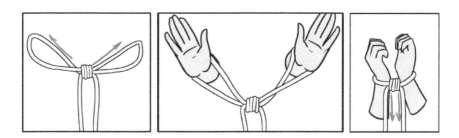

Then when you pull the two loops together outwards you will have what you see on the left hand side. Now you can place it around the wrists of your model and tighten. This is an excellent wrist tie to start out with in your art form.

Hand tying "stirrup" (second variant)

Take your rope and in the middle create a loop. Then pull the rest of the length of rope through the loop. After that, you'll want to bring the rope down and through again so as the palm side has four visible rope lengths as you see on the right hand side.

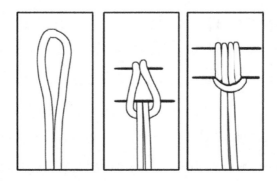

Now you will want to double up your loop as seen on the left. Then taking the ends of the rope you'll push it through the hole and then pull it all the way through as you'll see below.

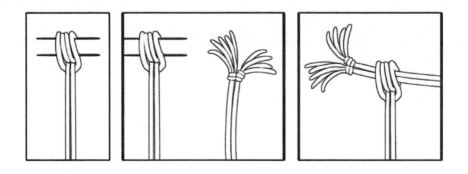

There you'll have the loop with your knot. The braid on there can be used to tighten it up around your models wrist as you see in the final image.

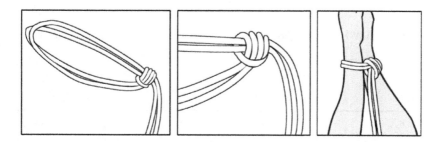

You can tighten it as much as you need, but exercise caution and communication with the model that you've chosen.

Wrist knot "chain"

With this next one you have a simpler approach for a similar type of wrist knot. Take the rope and create a U shape as seen on the left. Then as done in the middle you wits the rope so you have two big loops on either side. Then layer them on top of each other.

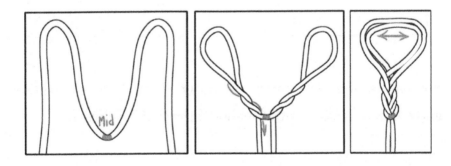

Insert your models arm through the two bigger loops. Then you'll pull the rope tight and it creates a strong knot and bond. For style and appearance you'll want to position it under the arm along the wrist as such in the right side image.

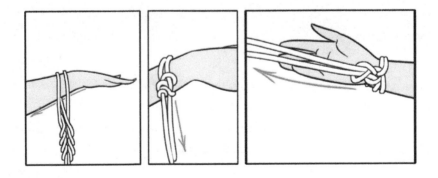

Arm knotting "rat-tail stopper"

This next knot we are going to look at is a more technical one. It involves actually tying up the whole arm and knotting it along the under arm. It looks great and it's a fantastic technique to utilize.

Take the ends of your rope into your hand as seen above. Then grab the rope and get it bent in the middle and then hold it in a loop. Follow the ends of the rope through the big loop you just made.

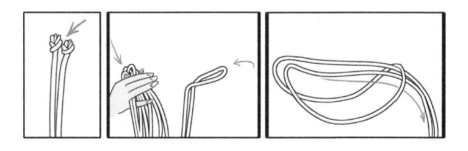

You are left with a loop as seen on the left hand side. Otherwise it's known as a larks head. Next you will want to put your arm through the loop at the apex of your shoulder and armpit. Then you will need to win the rope along your arm in a downward fashion. You'll want it to look similar to the image on the right.

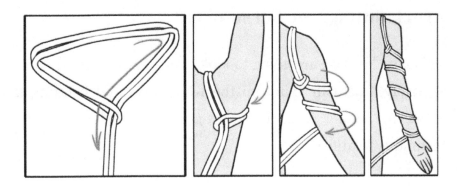

Take the rope and pull it back across itself in an X and then tuck it under the rope along your wrist then wrap it around and pull it to you going underneath the top you just wrapped.

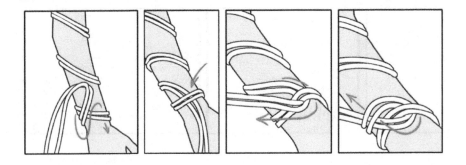

To keep the knot going, you pull the rope along your arm across the next wrap and then loop it under and then around over top of the rope body you just draped across. Then tuck it underneath the initial wrap that you pulled the rope across. You can see in the right hand image.

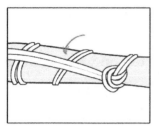 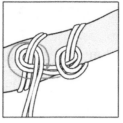 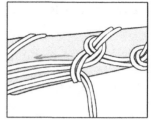

Then repeat that previous step for each wrap of rope that you come across as seen in the middle image. You should have 3 in total not including the first one done at your wrist.

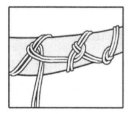 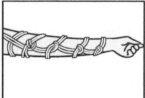 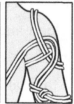 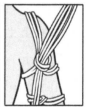

In order to finish the knot you will pass the rope underneath the loop on your shoulder and then loop it back through the larks head which will prevent it from cinching too tight! There you have it! Your first is more complex and elaborate knotting and tying experience.

Arm & neck tying "common whipping"

This is going to be another very complicated one, but again as well it is incredibly intriguing and the finished product looks great. This is one that starts out around the neck and then connects to a bind on both arms. It is a very restricting and fun technique that is favored in most circles of artistic Shibari.

Start out by folding the length of rope into halves and positioning the loop at the middle of the neck with the loop wrapped around as seen in the image. Then you'll want to tie a knot with the loop and main cord of rope on the back if the neck. You should be careful to not do it too tight and you should be able to fit at least two fingers between the rope itself and the flesh of your model.

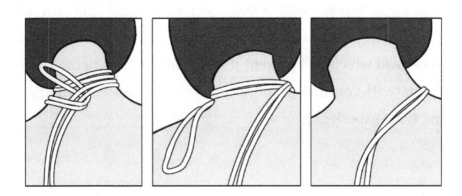

So now you'll be taking another length of rope and folding it in half. With this one you will take the main loop and wrap it around the loops and then again run the rope through the next loop made in a sort of weaving fashion seen in the second image. Continue that going back and forth, remembering to cinch it tighter each time and then, until you reach about midway down the arm.

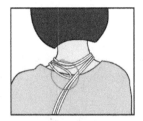 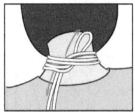 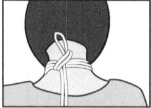

It should look as such from the other side, clean looking with no gaps between any ropes. Then in the next panel you see that we tie off the final loop in a simple knot and then it off to lock it with an over hand knot as seen on the right hand side.

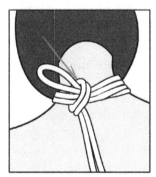 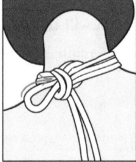 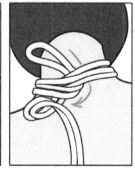

Here you will unite the neck rope with the arm rope down the back and then through the legs and up to the main portion of the arm rope. You'll want to connect the two of them with a Fisherman's knot to keep it nice and secure. Then if you have rope left over you can then tie another overhand knot below the bellybutton and loop the rope around itself for an aesthetic achievement to go the extra mile.

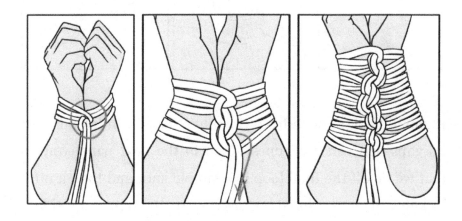

In order to remove the tie at the neck in times of discomfort or just ease of removal, you will then push the loop that sticks out, back in through the main knot as you see above in the three images.

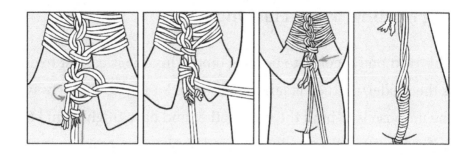

Then if you just pull on the newly loosened rope it should just come away easily, freeing your model from being tied at the neck. And then it's making the arms easier to remove as well. A very simple and delicate solution to the elegant and complex knotting structure you just went through, another example of the beauty of the craft.

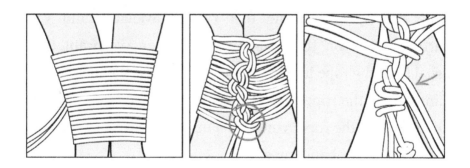

Leg binding "round lashing"

This next one is going to be a leg bind. This one is easiest to do if the model/partner is laid on their back or side. Either way, the purpose is to bind the leg together and have thigh bound to calf. This tutorial is easily reversed so you can practice it on both the right and the left leg.

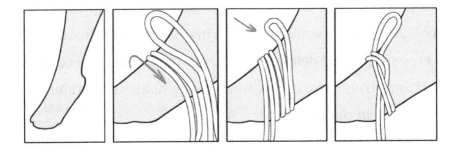

Start out by having the foot readily available and your partner/model on their back or side. Then you want to as usual have the rope folded into halves keeping the loop in your hand. Wrap the rope several times around the foot while still holding on to the rope. You'll then utilize the overhand knot as seen in the right hand image.

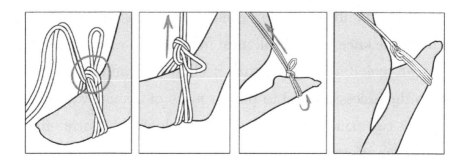

Now you'll pull up with the rope and then double not the rope around the main loop as seen in the second image. Now you want to pull the rope up so as you have the heel pressed to the model's butt as seen above, again you don't want it to be too tightly drawn.

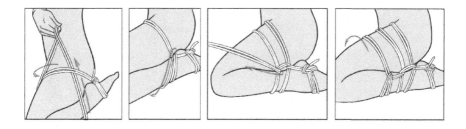

Now you'll want to wrap the rope around, over the thighs and then down and under the calf and then loop the rope underneath the main line. Take the rope back down again under the calf and then back around the top of the thigh back to the main line where you pull the rope under and through and then reverse it. Repeat that process until you get to the area just below your knee.

Here you will utilize your excellent over hand knot skills to tie it off at the knee. As you will most likely be left with extra rope, you can tuck it into the knotting itself or you can find a way to wrap the excess around to put on more of a show with it. In the last two panels you can see what it looks like form either side or the effort that goes into making the display.

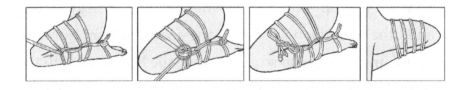

Hip tying "square lashing"

This next one is a hip and pelvic oriented tie and knot job. It is comprehensive but still simple, providing an excellent aesthetic look while being functional as a design.

Start out by making a small loop in the middle of the rope and then tying a double knot just below that. Then while holding that loop in place at the small of your models back, you'll want to pull the rest of the rope through the legs and tie another double knot but in front of you. Then have the model bring the knot down to their waist. There will be excess rope hanging down, which is a good thing.

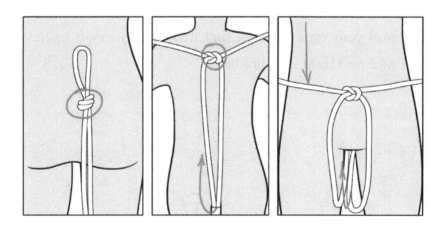

Pulling the rope back and then through the space below the loop that you knotted off, when pulled tight, should fit nice and snug around the crotch now.

The next step includes you pulling those ropes down and through the ropes in between the legs and then taking that back up to the loops on the hips and then repeating the process. You can see in the image on the right that you want it to be nice and tight.

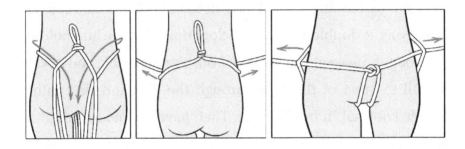

Take your rope and then pull it up underneath the loops you've already made but leaving a small loop held by your thumb. Then pull your rope through that little loop you left open and tug it nice and tight so it holds.

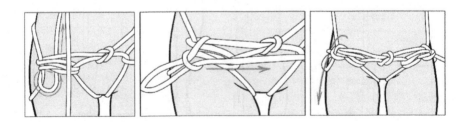

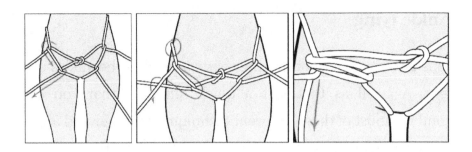

To finish it off you'll take the ropes and pull them back behind the models back and through that loop that you initially tied off. Then you'll tie it off at the loop and voila! You have your models hips and pelvis tied successfully.

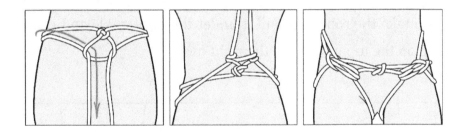

Ankle tying

This next one incorporates the wrists as well as the ankles and legs. As well as that just a quick reminder that you can combine most of these different techniques together and are in fact encouraged too. It's a great way to fine tune the craft and perfect the art form.

To start this one off you'll be binding your partner/model at the wrists using a simple wrist knot that you've learned already earlier in the book. Then you'll get them to kneel down and have their hands between their ankles as best as they can. Then take the rope and pull it under the right ankle and rest a loop on the top just above the right heel.

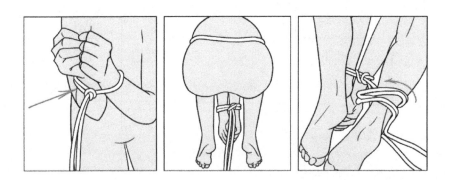

Take the extra rope section and pull it through the loop and them repeat what you did for the right ankle on the left ankle. After that you'll take the rope and pull it above and across the lower back of your partner over to the right hand side.

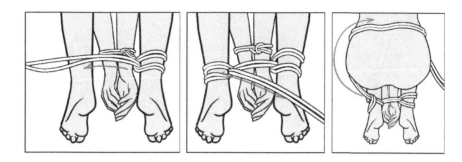

Now you'll be taking that rope you've draped across the lower back and tying an over hand knot at the right ankle. Simple quick knot, and then for style you'll wrap the rope around after securing the knot as far right as it will go.

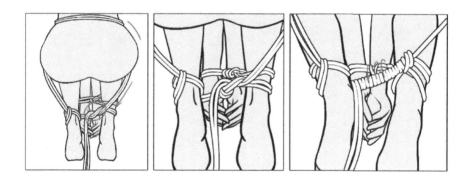

You'll do that same process for the left ankle, remembering to secure the knot and to tie off the last bit of rope after you've twirled it around the main line.

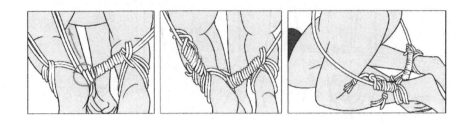

As I mentioned it binds the hands and the ankles and looks great. Remember though to always practice safety when doing these, especially the ones that completely limit the models range of motion. So exercise strict caution and even consider using a safe word.

Chest binding "figure 8 knot"

This next one is a two partner that starts out with a very simple chest bind and then leads into a wrist knot to tie it all together. Again, this is a thing that you can practice to learn how to do as well. Combine different knots with other knots or harnesses and explore what you're capable of and what you need.

To start off it's even fairly tame with a loop and then the rope being fed through that exact loop as seen in the middle image here right now.

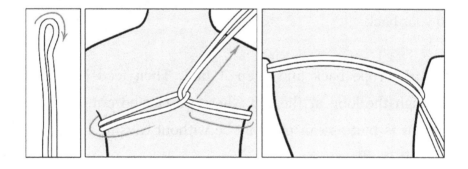

To continue you must then wrap the rope twice around the top above the bosom, and then once more below it. If you are using an exceptionally long piece of rope for this than you can even wrap the rope around a few more times each if you like. Then it's taking the last line of rope that it went across the front, and then loop it down through the lines of rope going across the body.

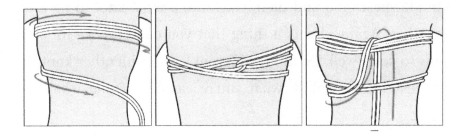

You want the rope you were just pulling to then be looped down but over the bottom loop so you create a cursive's' so to speak. Pull this loop tight and it should look like the pics in the middle. To keep the momentum going you'll then pull the tope to your back.

Pull the rope back and keep it taut. Then feed it up and through the loop at the top where we started out. Pull that until it is taut as can possibly be without causing harm, and then tie it off!

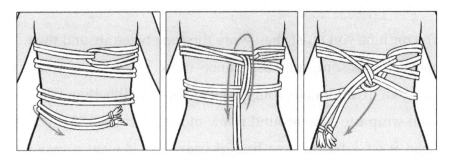

You can see the technique and how it's tied off. Then in the middle photo you can see how it looks once it's all finished, with the photo on the right being another representation of what the finished product looks like.

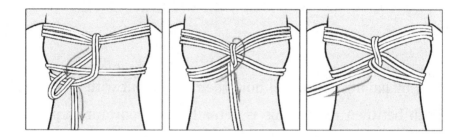

Chest & hand binding "figure 8 knot"

This is the second part to the last technique I showed you and is actually a direct add on. As I mentioned before a few times you can combine many of these different tying techniques with each other, but this is the first true example of what that would look like.

Start by having the model hold their hands out with a specific width between them. This is actually an important step that shouldn't be ignored. Now take the rope and lay it across the wrists with equal amounts of rope draped down either side. Then wrap the rope around the wrists a couple more times, still leaving equal amounts of unused rope on either side.

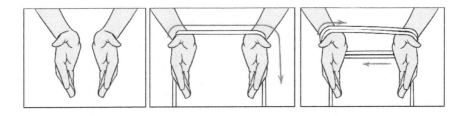

Keep wrapping it around until you've got around a total of five loops, two on either side of the original length of rope. For the next step you'll betting a knot underneath the bottom of the loops with the long lengths of ropes. Bring both ends up, one on either side and pull it tight.

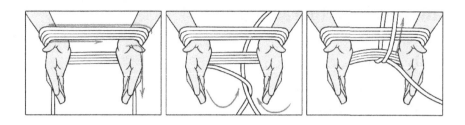

Loop the extra length in the centre with a loop on each side and keep it going until you have a nice looking coil, but remember to not cut off the circulation to the wrists. It's very important to keep that in mind. Once you have a great looking coil all done up its time to tie off the rope and admire your work. You can see how the two different rope techniques perfectly complement each other.

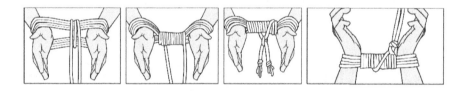

These have been some of the more basic and simple techniques in the knotting and tying for Shibari. With this book being a beginners guide into it we want to keep it fairly simple but at the same time you need something to challenge you. The last section of this book is 11 more different techniques of a slightly higher level. These next ones are also more full body, so they are perfect to learn so you can really become proficient in the craft.

Advanced Knotting & Tying

Body tying

To start we will drape the rope around the models shoulders like so. Then we will do knot it just above the breasts. This is where you need assistance from your model; they will need to hold the loop open slightly by pulling it from side to side. They will have to keep doing this as well while you tie a knot at the back.

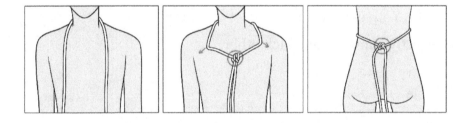

Next you will bring the lengths from behind around to the front and hook them on either side of the loop that the model was holding open for you. Pull it nice and tight as well, and then make sure you also do knotting that at the back too.

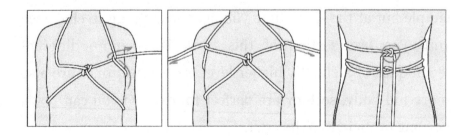

Now things will start to look somewhat complicated but don't worry I will explain you through the best I can. So now you take the rope and on either side you loop it up underneath the neck hole and create two big loops on either side. Pull them down as you see in the middle image. Then take the lengths from either side and run it through the opposing loop on both sides, as you see it in the image on the right.

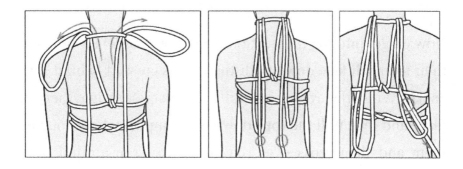

Pull it together nice and firmly so you get a lot of your length back from the rope. Then you'll want to run that rope length under the lower loops creating two new loops again as you did with it before hand.

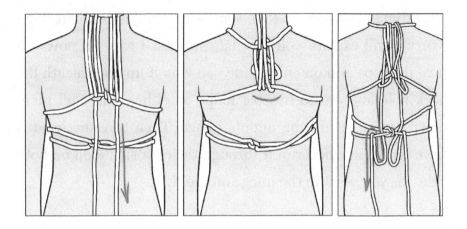

Now we get into the fun portion. Have your model lay down on their stomach face down with their arms crossed behind their backs. Wind the ropes around the wrists securing them in place and then pull the rope down to the ankles where you part them and then cross over the ankles to wrap around them several times.

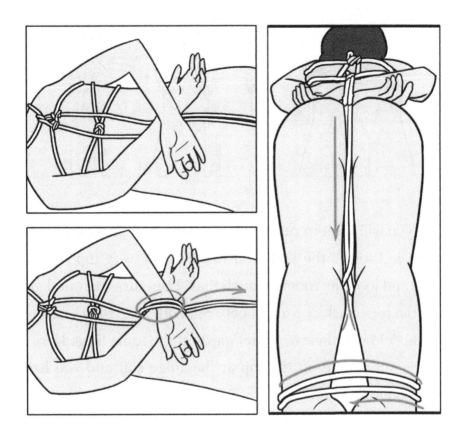

As you can see in the left image the ankles are wrapped, and then we wrap around the middle of the ankles to create a nice bind on them to keep them secure. You will now want to tie off the rope in the middle.

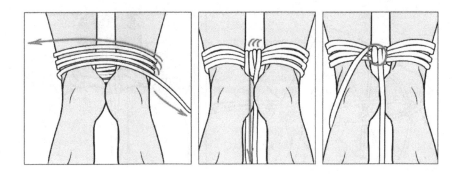

Now you will want to run that long length of rope back up their spine and locate the knot you made at the very top of their back, and loop the room through that. Then turn it around and pull the rope back down and between both feet while you have the model bend their legs backwards at the same time. Here is where you can tie off the top at the ankle cuff and you have your bonded model.

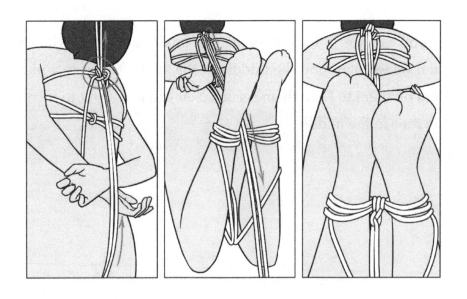

This is another one of those positions that because it's full bodies you need to put safety first and consider what could go wrong in any instant. Bond safely!

Double loops "bowline"

This one starts off with some off model designing first before we can get to them. Start out by making a double loop on the floor or any surface you have available.

Pull the double loop outwards into a bow which will knot it nicely as well. Now you get to put it onto your model. Get the, to put an arm in each loop so that the knot is entered on their mid back.

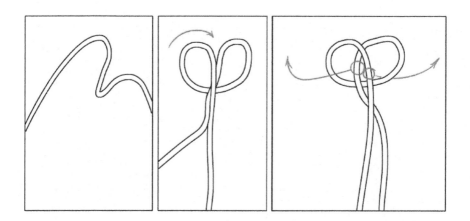

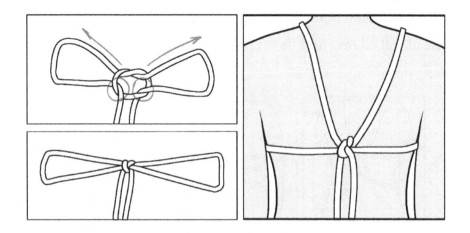

Take the rope and make another loop in your hands, then pull rope through enough so you can create two bigger loops. Pull it tight as well so it's cinched up with the main knot in the mid back.

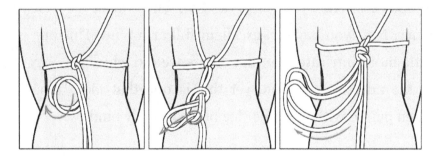

Get the model to put their arms through the new loops and place them around the mid arm mark, the biceps. If you pull on the free pieces of rope it should tighten up to be a nice bind. You can then repeat those steps several more times or as many as you'd like depending on how much rope you have available. The more you repeat the step the more interesting the pattern is. For the sake of this example we did three. One at the biceps, one at the elbows and then another at the wrists.

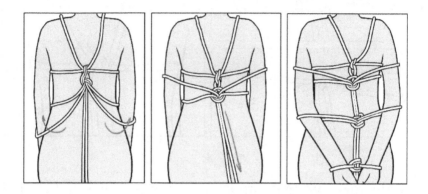

Now to finish it off, we take the long lengths of unused rope and wrap it around the lowermost rope bond, enough to make it look nice. Then you get to tie it off with whichever knot you fancy. Now you have an excellent full arm bind. This one is a little more intricate than the others we did which are why it's in the advanced section, yet this is one that looks amazing when paired with any other leg binds or body binds.

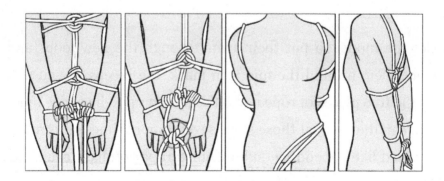

Body tying "fisherman's knot"

Again we have another one that starts with draping the rope around the neck at the halfway point of the rope itself. You will need the models help here with this one. For starters they will need to hold the rope at the collar bone level while you cross the ropes around the back at the spine. Loop the ropes back around and get the models help again to hold them in place while not dropping the placement of the ropes at the collar bone either.

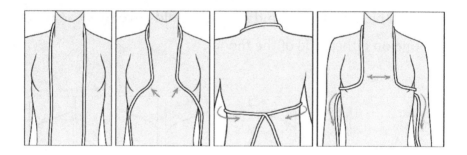

Take the rope being held in the right hand of the model and have it fed through both of the L shapes on the collar bones and then carry the rope around to the back.

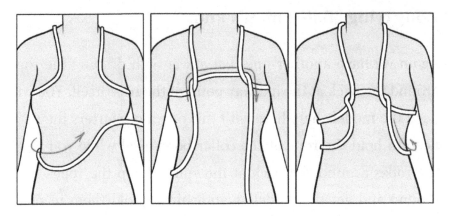

Here you are going to repeat the step you just did but this time using the left hand sided rope and going through two new L shapes that you've made just below the breasts. Again that rope will be fed back around so you should have two lose ropes still one on either side of the model.

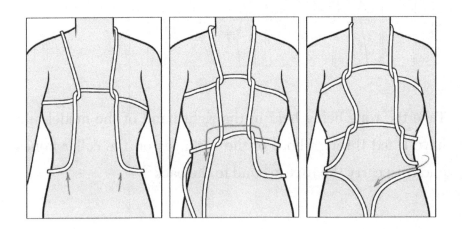

You can see what the back looks like during the process of this as well. Then as you've done a couple times already you will make the L shapes again on either side and then loop through.

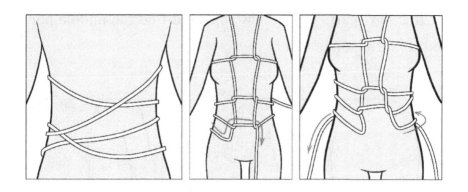

Keep the patterns going until you've reached around the hip area. That is where we begin the final steps for this specific technique. You can see a very cool and interesting pattern that's evolved.

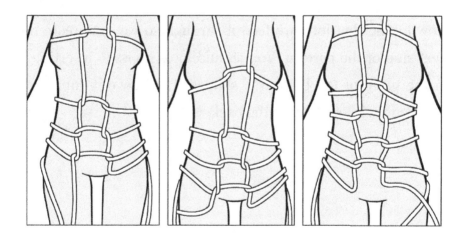

Now you are going to tie off the ropes at the back but you'll want to have the model holding the final two L shapes at the front down at the top of the pelvis to keep the tension accurate for this next part. Take a new rope and find the middle point and create a loop in hand.

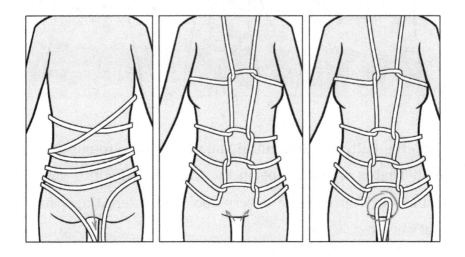

Now taking that loop we feed it through so we can create the next step of the pattern. You should have no issue inserting it in the place of the bottom L shapes. They have it run down between their legs and up the back.

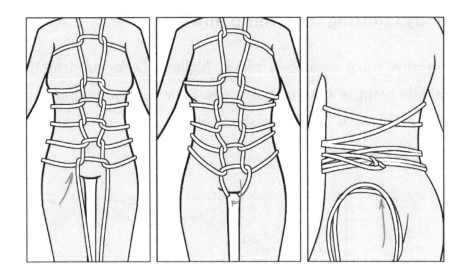

Once run up the back you'll want to loop it through the neck line that you started with and tie it off with an overhand hook. Now for aesthetic appeal we are going to wrap that length of rope we just led up the back with the remainder of the excess rope. Once that is done, tie it off and admire the finished product.

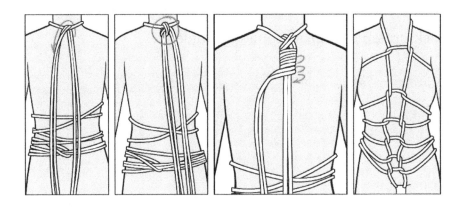

Body knotting "overhand bow"

For this you'll want two ropes. Make a Larks head at the middle point of both of the ropes. Slide an arm within each loop and have it rest at the shoulder sort of where a backpack would hang.

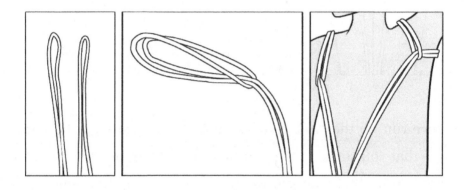

Now you will want to tie a nice sturdy knot in the middle of your chest. You can use any knot, though the one depicted is the one you've practiced a lot by now, the overhand knot. Once that is complete you will want to run the ropes behind your back, crossing them at around the middle.

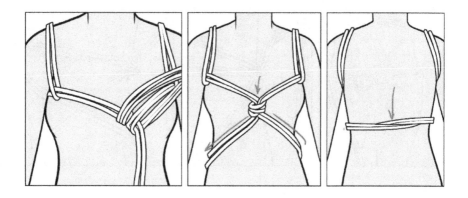

Pull the ropes to the front again and then tie them off once more, this time at your navel, again with whatever knot pleasures you. Then again you will run the ropes behind you to cross over one another, though this time down around your hips.

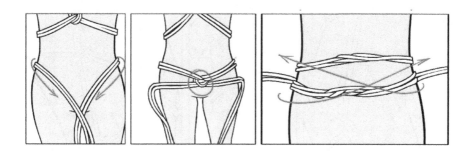

Once you have the ropes crossed at the back, taking one of the ropes run it inside your thigh and then back around the thigh just below your butt, it should create an X.

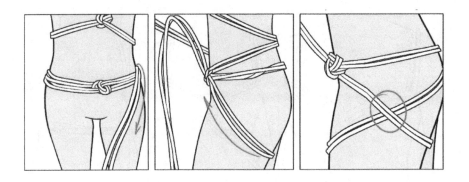

Where you have that X shape you'll want to create another thing you've gotten accustomed to, a hitch. They create another at each point that the rope crosses another line. This will finish off at the first larks head you tied around the shoulder.

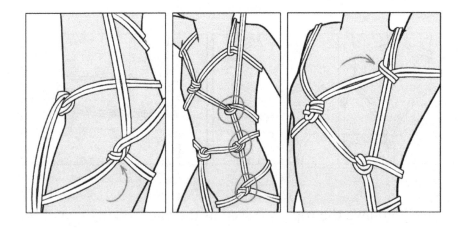

Now do the other side. You'll start with taking the rope and running it underneath the hitch you made on your waist, run the rope back along and then down through the inner thigh as well. Here you just need to follow the previous steps with the hitches and such, before you can call it totally finished.

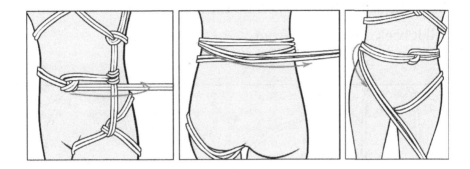

Now assuming you have no extra rope once all is said and done, then you're finished! However, if you do, you will take what you have and tie it off just behind your neck, leaving you with an excellent full torso bind that looks great and is something you don't actually need anyone help with when creating. It can be a totally solo affair.

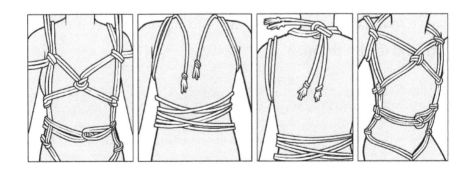

Back tying "cow hitch"

Here we start with the rope draped at its middle point across the neck. Bring the rope behind the back and cross it, and then pull it back out into the front.

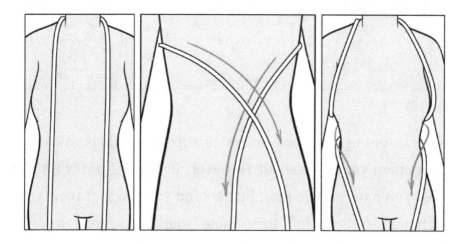

You then will need to put the rope through between the legs and tuck two larger loops on either side of the model. Once you've made those loops, take the end of the rope you made it with and feed it through.

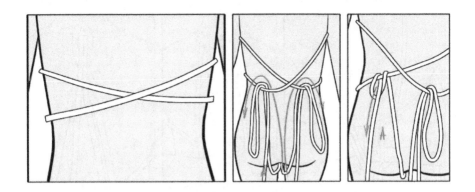

Once you've pulled the new loops taut, you get the person to put their hands behind their back and loop some of the excess rope around their wrists. Then in the next and last step just up above ups feed the extra rope through a couple more loops you've made and pull it tight.

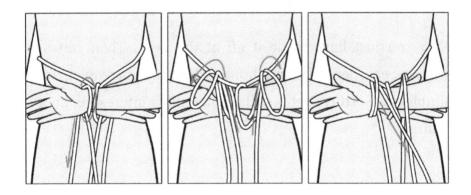

Pay attention to the ropes that are layered over each wrist. Then you will want to cinch it nice and tight and then make a nice firm knot between their two lengths of rope.

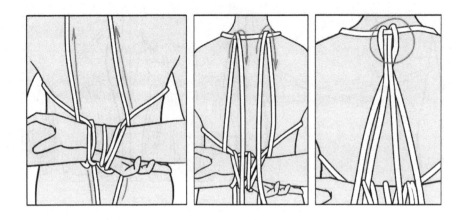

After tying off the knot, you'll need to take the ropes and feed them upwards just underneath the bound arms and then through the neck whole loop you started out with. As well create a loop for them so they can tighten up and secure the wrists and neck.

Now you just have to tie it off at the neck. Then you have another excellent tie and bond. This one has much more simplistic overtures yet is still an incredibly interesting knot to utilize.

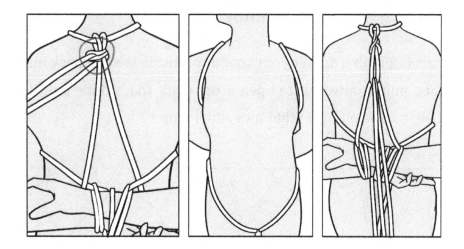

Binding "constrictor knot"

Start out with a double coin knot at or just below the neck line. Then pull it outwards to open it up. Once that's done pull the rope in on itself to get that nice small loop.

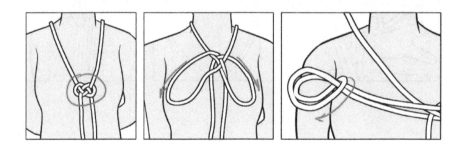

Your model will put their arms through those smaller holes, keeping their arms nice and secured. Now you will need to go through the 1-5 steps in order to create a nice pattern. For our example we did it the one time at the collar bone. Another time we did just below the bust of the model, and then for the last one it's placed just below the navel.

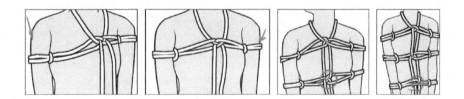

Once you have the pattern on the front locked down, you'll need to feed the ropes down between the legs and up along the back/spine and into the neck whole line you first made. Here is where the ropes get split in two to handle their own job which is to tuck it through the top most arm loop.

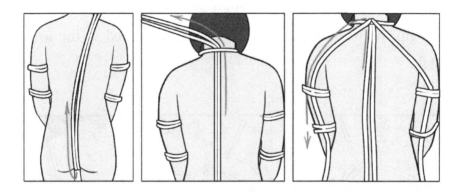

Now for the last couple steps, they are based almost purely in style. As you cross the rope back, forth time to create an excellent pattern. From there you will tie it off at the bottom and call it finished! Another masterpiece!

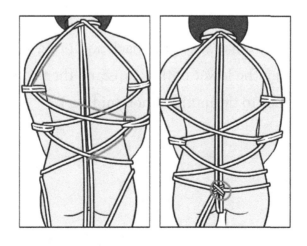

Coin knot "double overhand"

Now we have another one with humble double coin knot beginnings. They then get spread into four loops that are pulled open. Also the loose ropes get pulled between the legs and up the back, make sure there is a knot tied at the lower back.

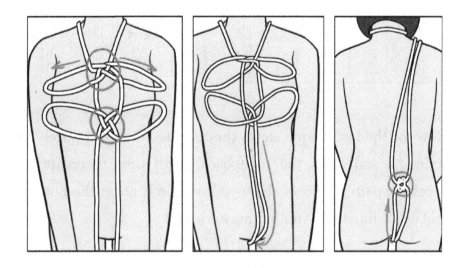

Take those ropes that are at the back and bring them forward to feed through the lower of the loops and then run them back behind the back to tie another knot, mid back.

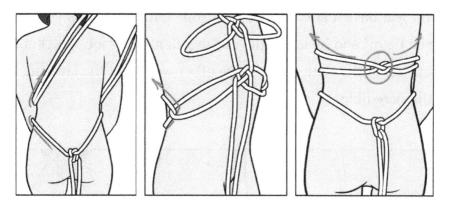

Once that mid-back knot is tied, run the ropes to the front again and through the upper loops, make sure to pull it taut. Then you run the rope under the armpits and push it through the neck hole and then pull tight.

You will take the left rope and run it through the mid back ropes as well as back through itself creating a knot that you can see in the images above. You will then do that exact same thing for the right hand side.

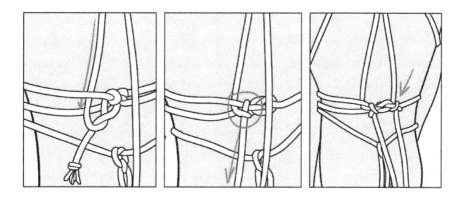

You will have a small amount of rope left over which you can then tie off and be left with your excellent tying job. The knots here are easier than some of the other works yet the layering is still incredible.

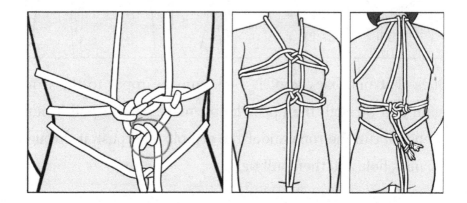

Tying "ashley stopper knot"

You'll be taking your rope, halving it and creating a loop. You'll run the rope behind the back and then pass the rope through the loop to make a giant larks head. You'll position that at the back but have the rope be across the upper chest.

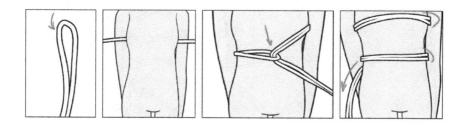

Taking the rope you'll run it around your body several times, as you can see. Them you will run the rope around the inner thigh and up the butt it to cross the waist loops. You'll want to hook those two together and then draw the rope across just under the belly button and to the back.

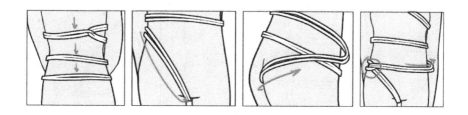

Then you'll take that rope and run it across the left butt cheek now and then between the legs and up the front. Your butt will now have a supportive V shape on it. Then you will take the rope upwards to your hip and hook it much like the last set of steps when you hooked the rope at the hip on the other side. From there you'll take the rope and loop it under the right butt cheeks line of rope and hook it upwards with a hitch.

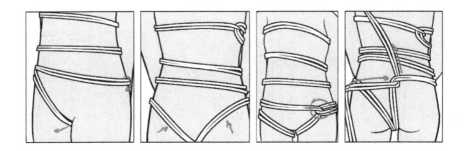

You'll hitch your way up the back with the rope, securing a strong and sturdy hitch at the middle of every loop. Here is where you will now separate the ropes having them pass one over each shoulder.

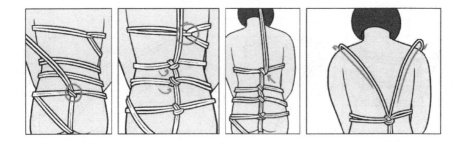

The separate strands of rope will meet at the middle of the first torso wrap and then you can start to hitch your way all the way down the front side. When you've reached the bottom you'll pass the rope down through the legs and across the centre of the groin in order to pass it back over the right butt cheek in order to bring back the supportive V it once enjoyed.

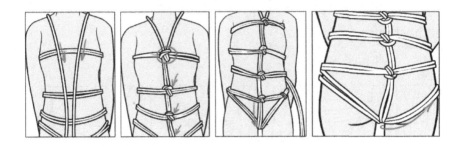

Then all that's left is to tie it off and hide any extra rope you have left over, you can either tuck it under a loop or you can wrap it or even cut it. Either way, once tied off, you have this amazing full body tie that looks incredible.

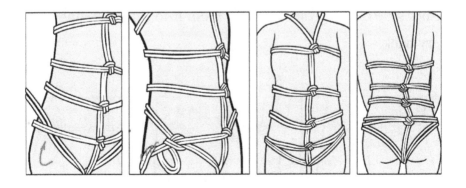

Difficult tying

Have you a loop in the middle of a length of rope. Place that rope around the waist with the loose ends getting fed through the loop. Wrap that around the body once more, and then feed the rope through the middle of the two ropes that are on the farthest left.

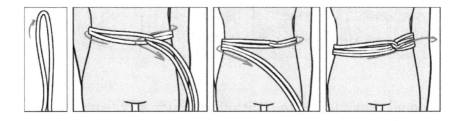

Take the loose ends you just wove through the left and then loop them over and weave them through the right side as well. Then part those strands and run them through the legs on either side of the groin and tuck them into the waist line at the very back.

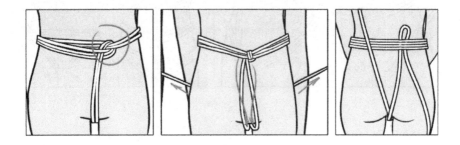

Feed the rope through its own little loops you've created on either side of the middle of your back, and pull it tight. Now you will need your model/partner to put their hands in prayer position behinds the back of their head.

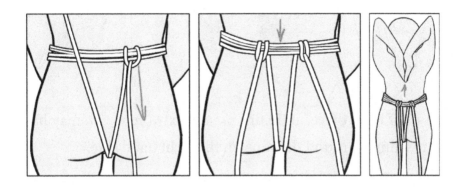

Take another rope and weave a loop around the wrists three or four times. Leave a nice enough loop at the top and then tie it off.

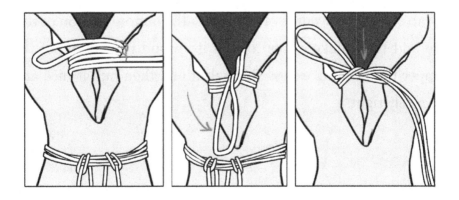

Take the rope and wrap it around the front, it should go across their biceps as well as in between their teeth. They push it through the loop you left available at the wrists.

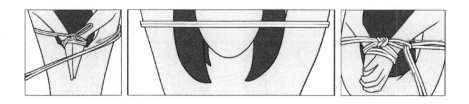

Tie it off right there, and burn off any extra rope you may have by twirling it around the rope on the right hand side.

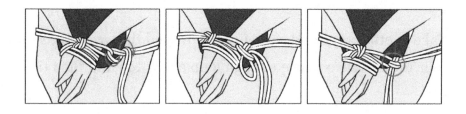

Grab one of the strands of rope from the bottom section of this tie and then make a loop out of it around the middle of the upper tie. Feed its excess through it and then pull it nice and securely tight.

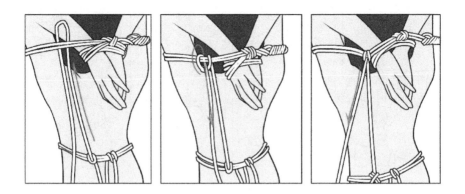

Take that bit of rope down to the waist section and then loop it through and tie it off. You will want to repeat that process with the other side as well to make it even and symmetrical.

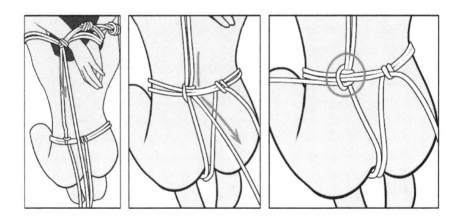

Here you can see that any excess rope can get dealt with by winding it around the preexisting rope. What you are left with is a beautiful display of craftsmanship and artistic expression.

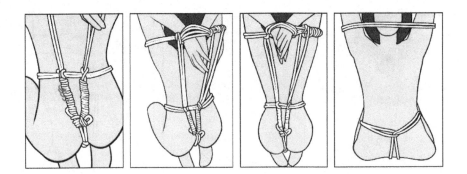

Knotting rope

Last but not least, number 11. This one is less of a useful tie and bind but more of a useful trick for storing and placing your rope somewhere. Why is it in the advanced section then? Because taking care of your rope is an incredibly important concept to understand. That rope is the tool of the trade, the paintbrush to the canvas of Shibari. Check out the technique below.

Grab the ends of the rope and then let there be a distance of almost two feet from the ends to where you pinch it with your other hand. Rotate it back and forth to collect and wrap up the rope.

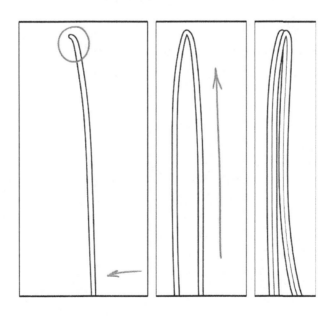

With the ends being the starting point, you'll eventually get to the loop at the very end. Hold the middle of your rope bundle and pull the end with the loop out a bit. Then you can use that to start wrapping around the body of rope.

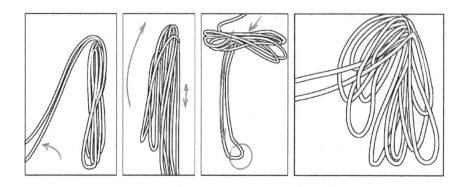

As you can see you want to wrap fairly tightly but allow a touch of slack for any adjustments needing to be made. Once you reach near the end, with one hand hold the coil and bundle, and with the other fold the loop in half and feed it into the end of the bundle. Then slide the coil up creating a sort of lock for the rope that keeps it from falling apart.

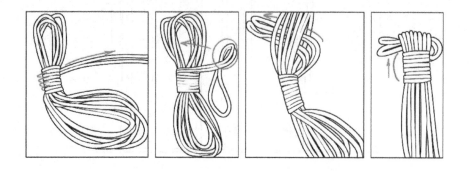

Then should you need to release it with ease, you need just pull out the loop hold it tightly, and then toss the rope and it unravels in an instant.

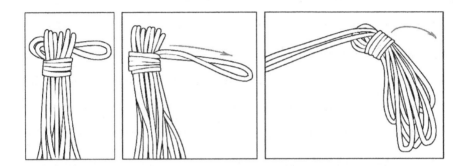

That sums up the best and boldest beginner moves and techniques to be taught for Shibari in tying and knotting.

Conclusion

You have now learned more than enough skills and techniques and talents to start practicing Shibari either on your own or with a trusted partner or friend. This is an art form that requires patience, skill, practice as well as immense caution. If there's one thing that hasn't been stressed enough in this book yet, it will be careful. You never know what could happen. Make a safe word; keep scissors or something sharp nearby if you can't untie the rope during an emergency. Either way, play it safe, but most importantly have fun and enjoy it. It is an art form, but it's also an exercise. Make it your own, find ways to explore and learn everything you can about it. Don't be afraid to share it with people or to embrace it as your passion.

Thank you for reading and best luck on your adventures!

Made in the USA
Las Vegas, NV
02 November 2023